The Healing Breast Cancer Cookbook

Nurturing Recipes for Renewal, Resilience, and Recovery

Dr. Leah Smith

CONTENTS

INTRODUCTION

Welcome to the Healing Breast Cancer Cookbook. This cookbook is a collection of nurturing recipes designed to support women with breast cancer during their treatment and recovery journey.

The healing power of food cannot be understated, and we believe that the right nutrition can help women overcome some of the challenges of breast cancer treatment.

In this book, you will find a variety of recipes that are both nourishing and delicious, and that are tailored to meet the specific nutritional needs of women with breast cancer. From energizing smoothies to comforting soups and stews, satisfying salads to wholesome entrées, and even delicious desserts, our recipes are designed to help you stay healthy, strong, and positive throughout your journey.

We understand that cooking and meal planning can be challenging during cancer treatment, which is why we have included helpful tips and resources to make things easier for you. We hope that this cookbook will not only provide you with nutritious and delicious recipes but also offer you comfort, inspiration, and a sense of community.

The Power of Food in Breast Cancer Treatment and Recovery

Breast cancer is a challenging and life-changing experience that can take a toll on both your physical and emotional well-being.

Treatment can cause a variety of side effects, including nausea, fatigue, loss of appetite, and changes in taste and smell.

Eating a healthy and balanced diet can help you manage these side effects, reduce inflammation, and support your immune system.

In addition to its physical benefits, food can also have a profound impact on your emotional health.

Cooking and sharing meals with loved ones can provide a sense of comfort and connection, while nourishing yourself with wholesome and delicious food can help you feel empowered and in control.

At The Healing Breast Cancer Cookbook, we believe that food is an essential part of breast cancer treatment and recovery.

Our recipes are designed to help you nourish your body and soul, so that you can feel your best during this challenging time.

How to Use This Book

This cookbook is designed to be a practical and user-friendly resource for women with breast cancer. Here are some tips on how to get the most out of it:

1. Read the introduction and the section on the power of food in breast cancer treatment and recovery.

   These sections will help you understand the importance of nutrition during cancer treatment and how the recipes in this cookbook can support you.

2. Browse the contents and select the recipes that appeal

to you. We have organized the cookbook into different categories to make it easier for you to find what you are looking for.

3. Use the bonus resources section to help you plan your meals and stock your kitchen. This section includes a breast cancer nutrition guide, a pantry essentials checklist, and meal planning tips and tricks.

4. Share your experience with us. We would love to hear from you about how these recipes have helped you during your breast cancer journey.

We hope that this cookbook will be a valuable resource for you during your breast cancer journey.

Remember to be kind to yourself and to nourish your body and soul with wholesome and delicious food.

Chapter 1

Conventional risk factors

Breast cancer is a complex disease with numerous risk factors, both modifiable and non-modifiable. Here are some of the traditional risk factors associated with breast cancer:

1. Age: As women age, their risk of developing breast cancer increases. Most breast cancers occur in women over the age of 50.

2. Gender: Breast cancer is more common in women than men. Men can also develop breast cancer, but it is rare.

3. Family history: Women who have a first-degree relative (mother, sister, or daughter) who has been diagnosed with breast cancer have a higher risk of developing the disease.

4. Genetic mutations: Certain genetic mutations, such as BRCA1 and BRCA2, increase the risk of developing breast cancer.

5. Personal history of breast cancer: Women who have previously had breast cancer have a higher risk of developing a new cancer in the other breast or a recurrence of the original cancer.

6. Race and ethnicity: Breast cancer incidence rates vary among different racial and ethnic groups. For example, non-Hispanic white women have a higher incidence of breast cancer than Hispanic, African American, or Asian women.

7. Reproductive factors: Women who have had their first menstrual period before the age of 12, have not had children or have had their first child after the age of 30, and/or have gone through menopause after the age of 55 have an increased risk of developing breast cancer.

8. Hormone replacement therapy (HRT): Long-term use of HRT that combines estrogen and progesterone increases the risk of breast cancer.

9. Breast density: Women with dense breast tissue have a higher risk of developing breast cancer.

10. Radiation exposure: Women who have had radiation therapy to the chest for another condition, such as Hodgkin's lymphoma, have an increased risk of developing breast cancer.

It's important to note that having one or more of these risk factors does not necessarily mean that a person will develop breast cancer.

Likewise, not having any risk factors does not guarantee that a person will not develop breast cancer. Regular breast cancer screening and early detection are important for all women, regardless of their risk factors.

Chapter 2

New Risk Elements

In addition to traditional risk factors, there are several emerging risk factors for breast cancer. These include:

1. Environmental toxins: Exposure to certain environmental toxins such as pesticides, polycyclic aromatic hydrocarbons (PAHs), and polychlorinated biphenyls (PCBs) may increase the risk of breast cancer.

2. Night shift work: Working night shifts may disrupt the body's circadian rhythm and

lead to decreased melatonin production, which may increase the risk of breast cancer.

3. Sedentary lifestyle: Lack of physical activity and sedentary lifestyle may increase the risk of breast cancer.

4. Hormonal contraceptives: Some studies have suggested that long-term use of hormonal contraceptives may increase the risk of breast cancer.

5. Hormone replacement therapy: Use of hormone replacement therapy (HRT) after menopause may

increase the risk of breast cancer.

6. Alcohol consumption: Alcohol consumption, even in moderate amounts, has been linked to an increased risk of breast cancer.

It is important for breast cancer patients to be aware of these emerging risk factors and make lifestyle changes where possible to reduce their risk.

Chapter 3

Preventable Exposures

There are several avoidable exposures that have been linked to an increased risk of breast cancer in some studies. These include:

1. Alcohol consumption: Drinking alcohol, even in moderate amounts, has been associated with an increased risk of breast cancer. Women who consume three to six alcoholic drinks per week have a small increase in risk compared to nondrinkers, while women who consume more than six drinks per week have a higher risk.

2. Hormone replacement therapy (HRT): HRT is used to relieve symptoms of menopause, but it has been linked to an increased risk of breast cancer. The risk depends on the type of HRT, the duration of use, and the woman's age when she starts using HRT.

3. Obesity: Being overweight or obese increases the risk of breast cancer, particularly in postmenopausal women. This may be due to higher levels of estrogen in fat tissue.

4. Lack of physical activity: Women who are physically inactive have a higher risk of

breast cancer compared to women who exercise regularly. Exercise may reduce breast cancer risk by lowering estrogen levels.

5. Environmental pollutants: Exposure to certain environmental pollutants, such as pesticides, has been linked to an increased risk of breast cancer. However, the evidence is limited and more research is needed.

6. Smoking: Smoking has been linked to an increased risk of many types of cancer, including breast cancer. The risk may be higher in women who start smoking at an early

age or who smoke for a long time.

It's important to note that not all women who are exposed to these factors will develop breast cancer, and some women who develop breast cancer may not have been exposed to any of these factors.

However, reducing exposure to these avoidable risk factors may help lower the risk of breast cancer.

Chapter 4

Adequate and Effective nutrient Intake

Breast cancer patients need proper nutrition to help their body fight the cancer, rebuild tissue, and maintain strength during and after treatments.

Adequate nutrient intake can also help manage side effects of treatments such as nausea, fatigue, and weight loss. Below are some key nutrients and their importance for breast cancer patients:

1. Protein: Essential for rebuilding tissue damaged by cancer treatment and for

maintaining muscle mass. Good sources include lean meat, fish, poultry, beans, and dairy products.

2. Fiber: Helps maintain digestive health and prevent constipation, a common side effect of chemotherapy. Good sources include fruits, vegetables, whole grains, and legumes.

3. Vitamins and Minerals: Important for maintaining immune function and overall health. Some important vitamins and minerals include:

- Vitamin D: Helps with calcium absorption and bone

health. Good sources include sunlight, fortified milk and cereals, and fatty fish.

- Calcium: Helps build and maintain strong bones. Good sources include dairy products, leafy greens, and fortified foods.

- Iron: Important for maintaining energy levels and preventing anemia. Good sources include red meat, poultry, fish, beans, and fortified cereals.

- Vitamin C: Important for wound healing and immune function. Good sources include citrus fruits, strawberries, kiwi, and peppers.

- B vitamins: Important for energy metabolism and nerve function. Good sources include whole grains, meat, fish, and leafy greens.

4. Omega-3 Fatty Acids: Have anti-inflammatory properties and may help reduce the risk of breast cancer recurrence. Good sources include fatty fish, flaxseed, chia seeds, and walnuts.

5. Antioxidants: Help protect cells from damage and may reduce the risk of cancer recurrence. Good sources include colorful fruits and

vegetables, nuts, and whole grains.

Breast cancer patients should strive to eat a balanced diet that includes a variety of nutrient-dense foods. It's important to work with a registered dietitian to develop a personalized nutrition plan that meets individual needs and preferences. In some cases, dietary supplements may be recommended to address specific nutrient deficiencies.

Chapter 5

Insulin, Glucose, and Weight Monitoring

Glucose, weight, and insulin control are important factors for breast cancer patients as they have been shown to affect cancer growth and recurrence.

High levels of glucose in the blood can promote cancer growth, so it is important for breast cancer patients to maintain normal blood sugar levels through a balanced diet and regular exercise.

Weight control is also important as obesity has been linked to an increased risk of breast cancer and poorer outcomes for those who do develop the disease. A healthy diet and regular exercise can help breast cancer patients maintain a healthy weight.

Insulin is a hormone that helps the body use glucose for energy, but high levels of insulin in the blood have been shown to promote cancer growth.

To control insulin levels, breast cancer patients should limit their intake of high-glycemic index foods, which can cause spikes in blood sugar and insulin levels.

Instead, they should focus on eating a diet that is rich in fiber and low in refined carbohydrates. This can help keep blood sugar and insulin levels stable, which can in turn help to prevent cancer growth and recurrence.

Additionally, regular exercise has been shown to improve insulin sensitivity, which can help to keep insulin levels in check.

Chapter 6

Enhancing Immunity

Maintaining a strong immune system is crucial for breast cancer patients, as it can help improve treatment outcomes and reduce the risk of infection. Here are some ways to nourish immunity:

1. Eat a balanced and nutrient-rich diet: Eating a variety of fruits, vegetables, whole grains, lean proteins, and healthy fats can provide the necessary vitamins, minerals, and antioxidants to support a strong immune system.

2. Stay hydrated: Drinking plenty of water and other

fluids can help flush out toxins and keep the body hydrated, which is essential for proper immune function.

3. Manage stress: Chronic stress can weaken the immune system, so it is important to find healthy ways to manage stress, such as practicing mindfulness, meditation, yoga, or other relaxation techniques.

4. Exercise regularly: Exercise can help boost immunity by increasing circulation and reducing inflammation. Aim for at least 30 minutes of moderate exercise most days of the week.

5. Get enough sleep: Lack of sleep can impair the immune system, so it is important to get enough restful sleep each night. Aim for at least 7-8 hours of sleep per night.

6. Avoid smoking and excessive alcohol consumption: Both smoking and excessive alcohol consumption can weaken the immune system and increase the risk of infections and other health problems.

7. Talk to your healthcare team: Your healthcare team can provide guidance on specific ways to support your immune system during breast cancer

treatment and recovery. They may recommend supplements or other interventions based on your individual needs and health status.

Chapter 7

Breast cancer patients' Inflammation

Inflammation is a natural immune response that helps the body fight infections and heal injuries. However, chronic inflammation can have negative effects on the body and is linked to several diseases, including cancer.

For breast cancer patients, managing inflammation is an important aspect of their overall health and well-being. Some dietary and lifestyle strategies that can help reduce inflammation include:

1. Eat a diet rich in anti-inflammatory foods: This includes foods like fruits, vegetables, whole grains, nuts, seeds, and fatty fish. These foods contain nutrients like antioxidants, fiber, and omega-3 fatty acids that can help reduce inflammation.

2. Limit processed and refined foods: Processed and refined foods like sugary snacks, white bread, and processed meats can promote inflammation in the body.

   Limiting these foods and focusing on whole, minimally processed foods can help reduce inflammation.

3. Maintain a healthy weight: Excess body fat can contribute to inflammation in the body. Maintaining a healthy weight through a balanced diet and regular exercise can help reduce inflammation.

4. Get regular exercise: Exercise has been shown to have anti-inflammatory effects in the body. Aim for at least 30 minutes of moderate-intensity exercise most days of the week.

5. Manage stress: Chronic stress can also contribute to inflammation. Strategies like mindfulness meditation, deep

breathing, and regular exercise can help manage stress and reduce inflammation.

By implementing these strategies, breast cancer patients can help manage inflammation in their bodies and support their overall health and well-being.

Chapter 8

Diminishing Burden

Lowering your toxic burden can help reduce the risk of breast cancer, especially for those who may have a genetic predisposition or have been exposed to environmental toxins. Here are some keys to help reduce your toxic burden:

1. Avoid harmful chemicals: Minimize your exposure to harmful chemicals, such as pesticides, plastics, and synthetic fragrances. Choose natural and organic products whenever possible, and read labels to avoid harmful chemicals.

2. Clean up your diet: Choose a whole-foods based diet that emphasizes fruits and vegetables, and avoid processed and packaged foods that may contain harmful additives and preservatives. Focus on anti-inflammatory foods, including omega-3 rich foods, and avoid foods that are high in sugar and saturated fats.

3. Drink plenty of water: Staying hydrated helps flush out toxins from your body. Choose filtered water, and consider adding a slice of lemon or lime for extra detoxifying benefits.

4. Exercise regularly: Exercise helps improve circulation and detoxification, while also reducing inflammation. Aim for at least 30 minutes of moderate exercise each day, such as brisk walking, cycling, or swimming.

5. Get enough sleep: Sleep is essential for detoxification and repair of your body. Aim for at least 7-8 hours of sleep each night, and create a relaxing sleep environment that is free from distractions.

6. Manage stress: Chronic stress can increase inflammation and reduce your body's ability to detoxify. Incorporate

stress-management techniques into your daily routine, such as yoga, meditation, or deep breathing exercises.

By following these keys, you can help reduce your toxic burden and improve your overall health and well-being.

Chapter 9

Hormone Balance

Maintaining hormone harmony is crucial for breast cancer patients. Hormones such as estrogen can promote the growth of some types of breast cancer, so managing hormone levels is important in reducing the risk of recurrence.

Here are some tips for maintaining hormone harmony:

1. Eat a balanced diet: A diet rich in whole foods, including fruits, vegetables, whole grains, and lean protein sources, can help regulate hormone levels.

2. Exercise regularly: Physical activity can help regulate hormone levels and reduce stress, which can also impact hormone balance.

3. Maintain a healthy weight: Being overweight or obese can increase estrogen levels in the body, which can increase the risk of breast cancer. Maintaining a healthy weight can help keep hormone levels in check.

4. Manage stress: Chronic stress can affect hormone levels, so finding ways to manage stress, such as through meditation, yoga, or other

relaxation techniques, can be beneficial.

5. Consider hormone therapy: For some breast cancer patients, hormone therapy may be recommended to reduce the risk of recurrence. This may include medications that block the effects of estrogen or reduce estrogen production.

It's important for breast cancer patients to work closely with their healthcare team to develop a personalized plan for managing hormone levels and reducing the risk of recurrence.

Chapter 10
Nourishing Breakfasts

. Energizing Smoothies

Energizing smoothies are a great option for breast cancer patients as they can be an easy and delicious way to provide your body with the nutrients it needs to support your health and recovery. Here are some tips for making energizing smoothies for breast cancer patients:

Choose nutrient-dense ingredients: Start with a base of nutrient-dense fruits and vegetables like berries, kale, spinach, and avocado. These ingredients are packed with vitamins, minerals, and antioxidants that can support your immune system and overall health.

Add a protein source: Adding a source of protein to your smoothie can help to keep you feeling full and satisfied throughout the morning. Consider adding protein powder, Greek yogurt, or nut butter to your smoothie.

Include healthy fats: Adding healthy fats to your smoothie can help to keep you feeling full and satisfied, and can also support brain health and reduce inflammation. Consider adding ingredients like chia seeds, flaxseeds, or coconut oil to your smoothie.

1. Include healthy fats: Adding healthy fats to your smoothie can help to keep you feeling full and satisfied, and can also support brain health and reduce inflammation.

   Consider adding ingredients like chia seeds, flaxseeds, or coconut oil to your smoothie.

2. Avoid added sugars: Avoid adding sweeteners like sugar or honey to your smoothie, as these can cause a spike in

blood sugar levels. Instead, sweeten your smoothie naturally with fruits like bananas or dates.

3. Consider adding supplements: If your healthcare provider recommends it, consider adding supplements like probiotics, vitamin D, or omega-3 fatty acids to your smoothie.

Here is a simple recipe for an energizing smoothie for breast cancer patients:

Ingredients:

- 1 cup kale
- 1/2 cup frozen mixed berries

- 1/2 avocado
- 1 scoop vanilla protein powder
- 1 tbsp chia seeds
- 1 cup unsweetened almond milk

Directions:

1. Add all ingredients to a blender and blend until smooth.

2. Pour into a glass and enjoy immediately.

Remember, smoothies can be a great addition to a healthy diet, but should not replace whole foods or meals. Be sure to talk to your healthcare provider or a registered dietitian before making any significant changes to your diet.

• Protein-Packed Omelets

Protein-packed omelets are a healthy and nourishing breakfast option for breast cancer patients.

Omelets can be a great way to start your day with a balanced and satisfying meal that can provide you with the energy and nutrients you need to support your health and recovery.

When making protein-packed omelets, it's important to choose ingredients that are high in protein and nutrients while also being low in unhealthy fats and sugars. Here are some tips for making protein-packed omelets for breast cancer patients:

1. Choose high-quality protein sources: Consider using eggs, egg whites, or egg substitutes as the base of your omelet. Other protein sources like lean turkey or chicken breast, low-fat cheese, or tofu can also be added to provide extra protein.

2. Load up on veggies: Veggies like spinach, peppers, mushrooms, and onions can add flavor and nutrition to your omelet. These veggies

are packed with vitamins, minerals, and antioxidants that can support your immune system and overall health.

3. Use healthy cooking fats: When cooking your omelet, consider using a healthy cooking fat like olive oil or avocado oil. These fats are high in heart-healthy monounsaturated fats that can help to reduce inflammation and support overall health.

4. Limit added salt and unhealthy fats: Be mindful of added salt and unhealthy fats like butter or bacon that can

be added to omelets. These ingredients can be high in calories and saturated fat, which can increase inflammation and negatively impact your health.

Here is a simple recipe for a protein-packed omelet for breast cancer patients:

Ingredients:

- 2 large eggs
- 1/2 cup chopped spinach
- 1/4 cup chopped mushrooms
- 1/4 cup chopped red peppers
- 1/4 cup shredded low-fat cheese
- 1 tsp olive oil

- Salt and pepper to taste

Directions:

1. In a small bowl, whisk together the eggs and a splash of water.

2. Heat the olive oil in a small nonstick skillet over medium-high heat.

3. Add the spinach, mushrooms, and peppers to the skillet and sauté for 2-3 minutes until the veggies are tender.

4. Pour the egg mixture over the veggies and let cook for 1-2 minutes.

5. Add the shredded cheese to one side of the omelet, then use a spatula to fold the other

side of the omelet over the cheese.

6. Cook for an additional 1-2 minutes until the cheese is melted and the eggs are cooked through.

7. Serve immediately.

Remember, omelets can be a great addition to a healthy diet, but should not replace whole foods or meals. Be sure to talk to your healthcare provider or a registered dietitian before making any significant changes to your diet.

• Oatmeal and Porridge Bowls

Oatmeal and porridge bowls are a delicious and nutritious breakfast option for breast cancer patients.

Oats are a great source of fiber, which can help to support digestive health and regulate blood sugar levels.

They are also packed with important vitamins and minerals like iron, magnesium, and zinc that can support overall health and recovery. Here's a guide to making a healthy and delicious oatmeal or porridge bowl:

Ingredients:

- 1/2 cup rolled oats or steel-cut oats

- 1 cup water or milk of choice

- Pinch of salt

- Toppings of choice, such as fresh or dried fruit, nuts, seeds, honey, or nut butter

Directions:

1. In a medium-sized saucepan, bring the water or milk to a boil.

2. Stir in the oats and a pinch of salt.

3. Reduce the heat to low and let the oats simmer for 10-15 minutes, stirring occasionally,

until they are cooked to your desired consistency.

4. Remove the oatmeal from the heat and let it cool for a few minutes.

5. Add any toppings of your choice, such as fresh or dried fruit, nuts, seeds, honey, or nut butter.

Tips for making the perfect oatmeal or porridge bowl:

- Use rolled oats or steel-cut oats for the best texture and flavor.

- Use water or milk of your choice, such as almond milk or coconut milk, to add extra flavor and creaminess.

- Add a pinch of salt to enhance the flavor of the oats.

- Cook the oats over low heat to avoid burning or sticking to the pan.

- Add toppings of your choice to make the oatmeal more flavorful and satisfying.

Serving suggestion:

A healthy serving of oatmeal or porridge bowl for breast cancer patients should be about 1/2-3/4 cup of cooked oats or porridge, and should be served with a variety of toppings like fresh or dried fruit, nuts, seeds, and a drizzle of honey or nut butter. It's important to note that while oatmeal and porridge bowls can be a healthy and nutritious breakfast option, they should not be relied on as the sole source of nutrition for breast cancer patients. Be sure to talk to your healthcare provider or a registered dietitian before making any significant changes to your diet.

• Muffins and Breads

Muffins and breads can be a tasty and convenient breakfast option for breast cancer patients. When made with healthy ingredients, they can be a great source of fiber, protein, and important vitamins and minerals. Here's a guide to making a healthy and delicious muffin or bread:

Ingredients:

- 2 cups whole wheat flour or flour of choice
- 1/2 cup rolled oats
- 1/4 cup honey or maple syrup
- 2 teaspoons baking powder
- 1/2 teaspoon baking soda
- 1/2 teaspoon salt
- 1 cup milk of choice
- 2 eggs
- 1/4 cup coconut oil or other healthy oil
- 1 teaspoon vanilla extract
- Optional mix-ins, such as fresh or dried fruit, nuts, or seeds

Directions:

1. Preheat the oven to 350°F (180°C) and line a muffin tin or bread pan with parchment paper.

2. In a large mixing bowl, combine the flour, oats, baking powder, baking soda, and salt.

3. In another mixing bowl, whisk together the milk, eggs, honey or maple syrup, oil, and vanilla extract.

4. Pour the wet ingredients into the dry ingredients and mix until just combined.

5. If desired, add any mix-ins, such as fresh or dried fruit,

nuts, or seeds, and mix gently.

6. Pour the batter into the prepared muffin tin or bread pan.

7. Bake for 20-25 minutes for muffins or 40-50 minutes for bread, or until a toothpick inserted into the center comes out clean.

8. Let the muffins or bread cool for a few minutes before removing from the tin or pan.

Tips for making the perfect muffin or bread:

- Use whole wheat flour or flour of your choice for added fiber and nutrients.

- Use honey or maple syrup as a natural sweetener instead of refined sugar.

- Add rolled oats for added fiber and texture.

- Use a healthy oil, such as coconut oil, olive oil, or avocado oil.

- Add in any desired mix-ins, such as fresh or dried fruit, nuts, or seeds, for added flavor and nutrition.

Serving suggestion:

A healthy serving of muffin or bread for breast cancer patients should be about one medium-sized muffin or one slice of bread, and should be served with a variety of other nutrient-dense foods, such as fresh fruit, a source of protein (e.g. Greek yogurt, nut butter), and a source of healthy fats (e.g. avocado, nuts). It's important to note that while muffins and breads can be a healthy and convenient breakfast option, they should not be relied on as the sole source of nutrition for breast cancer patients. Be sure to talk to your healthcare provider or a registered dietitian before making any significant changes to your diet.

Chapter 11

Comforting Soups and Stews

• Hearty Chicken Noodle Soup

Hearty chicken noodle soup is a comforting and nutritious meal for breast cancer patients. It's packed with protein and vegetables, and the warmth and spices can provide soothing relief during treatment. Here's a guide to making a healthy and delicious chicken noodle soup:

Ingredients:

- 1 tablespoon olive oil

- 1 medium onion, chopped
- 3 cloves garlic, minced
- 2 medium carrots, chopped
- 2 celery stalks, chopped
- 8 cups low-sodium chicken broth
- 2 cups cooked shredded chicken
- 2 cups uncooked egg noodles
- 1 bay leaf
- 1/2 teaspoon dried thyme
- Salt and pepper to taste
- Optional garnishes, such as fresh parsley or lemon wedges

Directions:

1. In a large pot or Dutch oven, heat the olive oil over medium heat.

2. Add the onion and garlic, and sauté for 3-5 minutes, until the onion is translucent.

3. Add the carrots and celery, and continue to sauté for another 3-5 minutes, until the vegetables are slightly softened.

4. Add the chicken broth, shredded chicken, egg noodles, bay leaf, thyme, and a pinch of salt and pepper.

5. Bring the soup to a simmer, and let cook for 10-15

minutes, or until the noodles are tender.

6. Remove the bay leaf, and taste the soup, adding more salt and pepper if needed.

7. Serve the soup hot, garnished with fresh parsley or lemon wedges if desired.

Tips for making the perfect chicken noodle soup:

- Use low-sodium chicken broth to control the sodium content of the soup.

- Use cooked shredded chicken from a rotisserie chicken or leftover cooked chicken to save time.

- Use whole wheat egg noodles for added fiber and nutrients.

- Add in any desired vegetables, such as mushrooms or kale, for added nutrition and flavor.

- Add in herbs and spices, such as rosemary or ginger, for added health benefits.

Serving suggestion:

A healthy serving of chicken noodle soup for breast cancer patients should be about one to two cups, and should be served with a variety of other nutrient-dense foods, such as whole grain bread, a side salad, or a piece of fruit. It's important to note that while soup can be a healthy and comforting meal, it should not be relied on as the sole source of nutrition for breast cancer patients. Be sure to talk to your healthcare provider or a registered dietitian before making any significant changes to your diet.

- ## Creamy Tomato Basil Soup

Creamy tomato basil soup is a comforting and delicious meal that can be enjoyed by breast cancer patients during treatment. It's packed with nutrients and antioxidants, and the creamy texture and warm spices can provide soothing relief during a challenging time. Here's a guide to making a healthy and flavorful tomato basil soup:

Ingredients:

- 1 tablespoon olive oil
- 1 medium onion, chopped
- 3 cloves garlic, minced
- 2 cans diced tomatoes (28 oz total)
- 2 cups low-sodium chicken or vegetable broth
- 1/2 cup heavy cream
- 1/2 cup fresh basil leaves, chopped
- 1/2 teaspoon dried oregano
- Salt and pepper to taste

- Optional garnishes, such as croutons or fresh basil

Directions:

1. In a large pot or Dutch oven, heat the olive oil over medium heat.

2. Add the onion and garlic, and sauté for 3-5 minutes, until the onion is translucent.

3. Add the diced tomatoes (with their juice) and broth to the pot, and bring the mixture to a simmer.

4. Let the soup simmer for 20-25 minutes, or until the tomatoes have broken down and the flavors have melded.

5. Remove the pot from heat, and use an immersion blender or regular blender to puree the soup until smooth.

6. Stir in the heavy cream, chopped basil, oregano, and a pinch of salt and pepper.

7. Return the pot to heat, and let the soup simmer for another 5-10 minutes, until heated through.

8. Taste the soup, adding more salt and pepper if needed.

9. Serve the soup hot, garnished with croutons or fresh basil if desired.

Tips for making the perfect tomato basil soup:

- Use low-sodium broth to control the sodium content of the soup.

- Use fresh basil leaves for a bright and flavorful taste.

- Use an immersion blender or regular blender to puree the soup until smooth.

- Use heavy cream for a creamy and comforting texture.

- Add in any desired vegetables, such as carrots or bell peppers, for added nutrition and flavor.

- Add in spices, such as cumin or red pepper flakes, for added depth of flavor.

Serving suggestion:

A healthy serving of tomato basil soup for breast cancer patients should be about one to two cups, and should be served with a variety of other nutrient-dense foods, such as a side salad, a piece of whole grain bread, or a piece of fruit.

It's important to note that while soup can be a healthy and comforting meal, it should not be relied on as the sole source of nutrition for breast cancer patients.

Be sure to talk to your healthcare provider or a registered dietitian before making any significant changes to your diet.

. Butternut Squash Soup

Butternut squash soup is a delicious and nutritious dish that can be enjoyed by anyone, including breast cancer patients. It is rich in vitamins A and C, fiber, and antioxidants, which can help to boost the immune system and support overall health. Here's a well-detailed and comprehensive note on how to make butternut squash soup:

Ingredients:

- 1 medium-sized butternut squash, peeled and cubed
- 1 large onion, chopped
- 2 garlic cloves, minced
- 4 cups of chicken or vegetable broth
- 1 cup of coconut milk or heavy cream
- 2 tablespoons of olive oil
- 1 tablespoon of ground cinnamon
- Salt and pepper to taste

Instructions:

1. Heat the olive oil in a large pot over medium heat.

2. Add the chopped onion and minced garlic, and sauté until the onion becomes translucent.

3. Add the cubed butternut squash to the pot and stir to combine with the onion and garlic.

4. Sprinkle the ground cinnamon over the squash and stir to combine.

5. Pour the chicken or vegetable broth over the squash and bring to a boil.

6. Reduce the heat to a simmer and let the soup cook for 20-25 minutes, or until the squash is tender.

7. Use an immersion blender or transfer the soup to a blender to puree until smooth.

8. Stir in the coconut milk or heavy cream, and salt and pepper to taste.

9. Serve hot, garnished with fresh herbs or croutons, if desired.

Serving:

- Serve the butternut squash soup hot in a bowl as a main dish or as a starter.

- Pair it with a slice of whole-grain bread or a salad for a complete and balanced meal.

- The soup can also be stored in an airtight container in the refrigerator for up to 3 days, or in the freezer for up to 3 months.

Overall, butternut squash soup is a delicious and healthy addition to any diet, including for those undergoing breast cancer treatment. It's easy to make, comforting, and packed with nutrients that can help support overall health and well-being.

• Beef and Vegetable Stew

Beef and vegetable stew is a hearty and comforting dish that is packed with protein and essential nutrients. It's a perfect meal for breast cancer patients who need a nutrient-rich diet to support their immune system during treatment. Here's a well-detailed and comprehensive note on how to make beef and vegetable stew:

Ingredients:

- 1 lb. beef stew meat, cubed
- 2 tbsp. olive oil
- 1 onion, chopped
- 2 garlic cloves, minced
- 4 cups of beef broth
- 2 large carrots, peeled and chopped
- 2 celery stalks, chopped
- 2 potatoes, peeled and cubed

- 1 can diced tomatoes
- 1 tsp. dried thyme
- Salt and pepper to taste

Instructions:

1. Heat the olive oil in a large pot over medium heat.

2. Add the cubed beef stew meat and brown on all sides.

3. Remove the meat from the pot and set aside.

4. Add the chopped onion and minced garlic to the pot and sauté until the onion becomes translucent.

5. Add the chopped carrots, celery, and potatoes to the pot and sauté for 5-7 minutes.

6. Add the beef broth, canned diced tomatoes, dried thyme, and salt and pepper to taste.

7. Bring the stew to a boil, then reduce the heat to a simmer and let it cook for 1-2 hours, or until the beef and vegetables are tender.

8. Adjust the seasoning if needed and serve hot.

Serving:

- Beef and vegetable stew can be served as a main dish, accompanied by a side salad or whole-grain bread.

- It can also be stored in an airtight container in the refrigerator for up to 3 days, or in the freezer for up to 3 months.

- When reheating the stew, add a little bit of water or broth to prevent it from becoming too thick.

Overall, beef and vegetable stew is a delicious and nutritious meal that can provide breast cancer patients with the protein and nutrients they need to support their health during treatment.

The dish is easy to make and can be customized to include other healthy vegetables, such as broccoli or spinach, to boost its nutritional value.

Chapter 12

Satisfying Salads

Kale and Quinoa Salad

Kale and quinoa salad is a tasty and healthy dish that is perfect for breast cancer patients. It's packed with protein, fiber, and essential nutrients that can support their immune system during treatment. Here's a well-detailed and comprehensive note on how to make kale and quinoa salad:

Ingredients:

- 1 cup quinoa, rinsed and drained
- 2 cups water

- 1 bunch of kale, stems removed and chopped
- 1 red onion, diced
- 1 red bell pepper, diced
- 1 avocado, diced
- 1/4 cup chopped fresh cilantro
- 1/4 cup olive oil
- 2 tbsp. apple cider vinegar
- 1 tbsp. honey
- 1 tsp. Dijon mustard
- Salt and pepper to taste

Instructions:

1. In a medium-sized pot, add quinoa and water and bring to a boil over medium heat.

2. Reduce the heat to low, cover the pot, and let the quinoa cook for 15-20 minutes or until tender.

3. Remove the pot from the heat and let it cool.

4. In a large mixing bowl, add the chopped kale, diced red onion, diced red bell pepper, and diced avocado.

5. Add the cooked quinoa to the bowl and mix everything together.

6. In a small mixing bowl, whisk together the olive oil, apple cider vinegar, honey, Dijon mustard, salt, and pepper to make the dressing.

7. Pour the dressing over the salad and mix everything together.

8. Add the chopped cilantro on top of the salad and serve.

Serving:

- Kale and quinoa salad can be served as a main dish or as a side dish.

- It can also be stored in an airtight container in the refrigerator for up to 3 days.

- When serving, add some additional protein sources such as grilled chicken or tofu to make it a complete meal.

Overall, kale and quinoa salad is a simple and nutritious dish that can provide breast cancer patients with the essential nutrients they need to support their health during treatment. The salad is easy to customize with other healthy vegetables, nuts, and seeds to increase its nutritional value.

• Greek Salad

Greek salad is a simple and delicious dish that is perfect for breast cancer patients who want a healthy and flavorful meal. Here's a well-detailed and comprehensive note on how to make Greek salad:

Ingredients:

- 1 head of romaine lettuce, chopped

- 1 cucumber, chopped

- 1 red onion, thinly sliced

- 1 red bell pepper, chopped

- 1/2 cup pitted Kalamata olives

- 1/2 cup crumbled feta cheese

- 1/4 cup extra-virgin olive oil

- 2 tbsp. red wine vinegar

- 1 tsp. dried oregano

- Salt and pepper to taste

Instructions:

1. In a large mixing bowl, add the chopped romaine lettuce,

chopped cucumber, thinly sliced red onion, chopped red bell pepper, and pitted Kalamata olives.

2. Add the crumbled feta cheese to the bowl.

3. In a small mixing bowl, whisk together the extra-virgin olive oil, red wine vinegar, dried oregano, salt, and pepper to make the dressing.

4. Pour the dressing over the salad and mix everything together.

5. Serve the Greek salad immediately.

Serving:

- Greek salad can be served as a main dish or as a side dish.

- It can also be stored in an airtight container in the refrigerator for up to 2 days.

- When serving, add some additional protein sources such as grilled chicken or chickpeas to make it a complete meal.

Overall, Greek salad is a healthy and flavorful dish that is packed with essential nutrients for breast cancer patients. The salad is easy to customize with other healthy vegetables, nuts, and seeds to increase its nutritional value.

Roasted Beet Salad

Roasted beet salad is a delicious and healthy salad that is perfect for breast cancer patients. Here's a well-detailed and comprehensive note on how to make roasted beet salad:

Ingredients:

- 4-5 medium beets, peeled and cut into wedges
- 1/4 cup extra-virgin olive oil
- 2 tbsp. balsamic vinegar
- Salt and pepper to taste
- 4 cups baby spinach
- 1/2 cup crumbled goat cheese

- 1/4 cup chopped walnuts

Instructions:

1. Preheat the oven to 400°F.

2. In a large mixing bowl, add the peeled and cut beet wedges, extra-virgin olive oil, balsamic vinegar, salt, and pepper. Toss everything together to coat the beets evenly.

3. Spread the beet wedges out on a baking sheet and roast for about 30-40 minutes, or until the beets are tender and lightly browned.

4. Remove the beets from the oven and let them cool for a few minutes.

5. In a large mixing bowl, add the baby spinach and toss it with a little extra-virgin olive oil and balsamic vinegar.

6. Add the roasted beet wedges, crumbled goat cheese, and chopped walnuts to the bowl.

7. Toss everything together to coat the salad ingredients with the dressing.

Serving:

- Roasted beet salad can be served as a main dish or as a side dish.

- It can also be stored in an airtight container in the refrigerator for up to 3 days.

- When serving, you can add some additional protein sources such as grilled chicken or tofu to make it a complete meal.

Overall, roasted beet salad is a delicious and healthy dish that is rich in antioxidants, fiber, and essential vitamins and minerals.

The salad is easy to prepare and can be customized with other healthy vegetables, fruits, and nuts to increase its nutritional value.

Avocado and Tomato Salad

Roasted beet salad is a delicious and healthy salad that is perfect for breast cancer patients. Here's a well-detailed and comprehensive note on how to make roasted beet salad:

Ingredients:

- 4-5 medium beets, peeled and cut into wedges
- 1/4 cup extra-virgin olive oil
- 2 tbsp. balsamic vinegar
- Salt and pepper to taste
- 4 cups baby spinach
- 1/2 cup crumbled goat cheese
- 1/4 cup chopped walnuts

Instructions:

1. Preheat the oven to 400°F.

2. In a large mixing bowl, add the peeled and cut beet wedges, extra-virgin olive oil, balsamic vinegar, salt, and pepper. Toss everything together to coat the beets evenly.

3. Spread the beet wedges out on a baking sheet and roast for about 30-40 minutes, or until the beets are tender and lightly browned.

4. Remove the beets from the oven and let them cool for a few minutes.

5. In a large mixing bowl, add the baby spinach and toss it with a little extra-virgin olive oil and balsamic vinegar.

6. Add the roasted beet wedges, crumbled goat cheese, and chopped walnuts to the bowl.

7. Toss everything together to coat the salad ingredients with the dressing.

Serving:

- Roasted beet salad can be served as a main dish or as a side dish.

- It can also be stored in an airtight container in the refrigerator for up to 3 days.

- When serving, you can add some additional protein sources such as grilled chicken or tofu to make it a complete meal.

Overall, roasted beet salad is a delicious and healthy dish that is rich in antioxidants, fiber, and essential vitamins and minerals.

The salad is easy to prepare and can be customized with other healthy vegetables, fruits, and nuts to increase its nutritional value.

Chapter 13
Wholesome Entrées

• Baked Salmon with Lemon and Dill

Baked salmon with lemon and dill is a nutritious and delicious dish that is easy to prepare. It is a great choice for breast cancer patients as it is high in protein, omega-3 fatty acids, and other essential nutrients that support healing and recovery.

Here is a detailed and comprehensive note on how to make baked salmon with lemon and dill:

Ingredients:

- 4 salmon fillets (6-8 ounces each)
- 1/4 cup olive oil
- 1/4 cup fresh lemon juice
- 2 tablespoons chopped fresh dill
- 2 cloves garlic, minced
- Salt and black pepper, to taste
- Lemon wedges, for serving

Instructions:

1. Preheat your oven to 375°F (190°C).

2. In a small bowl, whisk together the olive oil, lemon

juice, dill, garlic, salt, and pepper.

3. Place the salmon fillets skin-side down in a baking dish.

4. Pour the marinade over the salmon fillets, making sure they are well coated.

5. Cover the baking dish with aluminum foil and bake for 15-20 minutes or until the salmon is cooked through and flakes easily with a fork.

6. Remove the foil and broil the salmon for 2-3 minutes until the top is golden brown.

7. Serve hot with lemon wedges on the side.

Serving Diet: This dish can be served with a variety of sides, such as roasted vegetables, quinoa, or brown rice. It is also delicious when served over a bed of mixed greens or spinach. To make it a complete meal, be sure to include a source of carbohydrates, such as whole grains or starchy vegetables, and a variety of colorful fruits and vegetables.

. Turkey Chili

Turkey chili is a hearty and nutritious meal that is easy to prepare and perfect for a cold day. It is an excellent source of protein and fiber, making it an ideal meal for breast cancer patients. Here's a step-by-step guide on how to make turkey chili:

Ingredients:

- 1 lb ground turkey
- 1 tbsp olive oil
- 1 large onion, chopped
- 1 bell pepper, chopped
- 3 cloves garlic, minced
- 1 can of diced tomatoes
- 1 can of kidney beans, drained and rinsed
- 1 can of black beans, drained and rinsed
- 1 can of corn, drained
- 1 tsp cumin
- 1 tsp chili powder

- 1 tsp paprika
- Salt and pepper to taste
- 2 cups of water or chicken broth
- Optional toppings: shredded cheese, sour cream, chopped green onions

Instructions:

1. In a large pot, heat the olive oil over medium heat. Add the ground turkey and cook until browned.

2. Add the chopped onion, bell pepper, and garlic to the pot. Cook until the vegetables are softened.

3. Add the diced tomatoes, kidney beans, black beans, corn, cumin, chili powder, paprika, salt, and pepper to the pot. Stir well to combine.

4. Pour in the water or chicken broth, and bring the chili to a boil.

5. Reduce the heat to low and let the chili simmer for 30-45 minutes, stirring occasionally.

6. Serve the chili hot with your desired toppings.

Serving Diet:

This recipe serves about 6-8 people. Each serving contains approximately 250-300 calories. Turkey chili is best served with a side of brown rice or whole grain bread to make it a more filling meal. It can also be served with a green salad or steamed vegetables for added nutrients. This meal can be stored in an airtight container in the fridge for up to 4 days, or frozen for up to 3 months.

• Vegetable Stir-Fry

Vegetable stir-fry is a healthy and delicious dish that is easy to make and packed with nutrition. Here is a well-detailed and comprehensive note on how to make vegetable stir-fry:

Ingredients:

- 2 tablespoons of vegetable oil

- 1 red bell pepper, sliced
- 1 green bell pepper, sliced
- 1 yellow onion, sliced
- 1 cup of sliced mushrooms
- 1 cup of broccoli florets
- 1 cup of sliced carrots
- 2 garlic cloves, minced
- 1 tablespoon of soy sauce
- 1 tablespoon of hoisin sauce
- 1 teaspoon of honey
- 1 teaspoon of cornstarch
- Salt and pepper to taste

Directions:

1. Heat the vegetable oil in a large skillet over medium-high heat.

2. Add the sliced peppers and onion to the skillet and stir-fry for 3-4 minutes until they are slightly softened.

3. Add the sliced mushrooms, broccoli florets, and sliced carrots to the skillet and continue to stir-fry for an additional 3-4 minutes.

4. Add the minced garlic to the skillet and stir-fry for 30 seconds until fragrant.

5. In a small bowl, mix together the soy sauce, hoisin sauce,

honey, and cornstarch until well combined.

6. Pour the sauce over the vegetables in the skillet and stir-fry for an additional 1-2 minutes until the vegetables are coated in the sauce and it has thickened.

7. Season with salt and pepper to taste.

8. Serve the vegetable stir-fry hot with rice or noodles.

Serving diet: This vegetable stir-fry is a perfect dish for a healthy and balanced meal. It is low in calories and high in fiber, vitamins, and minerals, making it a great addition to any diet. It can be served with brown rice, quinoa, or whole-grain noodles for added nutrition.

• Beef and Broccoli Stir-Fry

Beef and broccoli stir-fry is a delicious and nutritious meal that can be enjoyed by breast cancer patients. It is a great way to get protein, fiber, and vitamins from the vegetables. Here's a well-detailed and comprehensive note on how to prepare beef and broccoli stir-fry:

Ingredients:

- 1 pound beef sirloin, thinly sliced

- 1/4 cup soy sauce

- 1 tablespoon cornstarch
- 1 tablespoon sesame oil
- 1 tablespoon vegetable oil
- 1 tablespoon minced garlic
- 1 tablespoon minced ginger
- 1 head broccoli, cut into florets
- 1 red bell pepper, sliced
- 1/2 cup beef broth
- 2 tablespoons oyster sauce
- Salt and pepper to taste

Instructions:

1. In a bowl, mix together the soy sauce, cornstarch, and sesame oil. Add the sliced

beef and toss to coat. Set aside.

2. Heat a large skillet or wok over medium-high heat. Add the vegetable oil and swirl to coat.

3. Add the minced garlic and ginger and stir-fry for 30 seconds or until fragrant.

4. Add the marinated beef to the skillet and stir-fry for 2-3 minutes or until browned.

5. Add the broccoli and red bell pepper to the skillet and stir-fry for 2-3 minutes or until tender-crisp.

6. Pour in the beef broth and oyster sauce and stir to

combine. Bring to a simmer and cook for 2-3 minutes or until the sauce has thickened.

7. Season with salt and pepper to taste.

8. Serve hot with brown rice or quinoa.

Serving diet: This recipe can serve 4 people. Each serving contains approximately 300-400 calories, 30 grams of protein, and 8 grams of fiber. It is a great main dish to serve for lunch or dinner. It can be paired with brown rice or quinoa for a complete meal.

Chapter 14
Delicious Desserts

• Chocolate Avocado Pudding

Chocolate Avocado Pudding is a delicious and nutritious dessert that can be enjoyed by breast cancer patients. This pudding is rich in healthy fats, fiber, antioxidants, and essential nutrients, and it is easy to make. Here's a well-detailed and comprehensive note on how to make Chocolate Avocado Pudding.

Ingredients:

- 2 ripe avocados

- 1/2 cup unsweetened cocoa powder
- 1/2 cup almond milk (or any other milk of your choice)
- 1/2 cup maple syrup or honey (adjust to taste)
- 1 teaspoon vanilla extract
- a pinch of sea salt

Instructions:

1. Cut the avocados in half and remove the pit. Scoop the flesh out into a blender or food processor.

2. Add the cocoa powder, almond milk, maple syrup or honey, vanilla extract, and sea

salt to the blender or food processor.

3. Blend or process the ingredients until smooth and creamy, scraping down the sides as needed.

4. Taste the pudding and adjust the sweetness if necessary. You can also add more cocoa powder for a richer chocolate flavor.

5. Transfer the pudding to individual serving dishes or a large bowl.

6. Chill the pudding in the refrigerator for at least 30 minutes before serving.

7. Garnish with fresh berries, sliced nuts, or shredded coconut before serving, if desired.

Serving: This recipe makes about 4 servings of chocolate avocado pudding. You can store any leftovers in an airtight container in the refrigerator for up to 3 days. This pudding can be enjoyed as a healthy and indulgent dessert, or as a snack or breakfast. It is also a great way to satisfy your chocolate cravings without consuming unhealthy ingredients like refined sugar or processed chocolate.

Fresh Fruit Salad

Fresh fruit salad is a refreshing and healthy dish that can be enjoyed as a snack or dessert. It's easy to prepare and can be customized to include your favorite fruits. Here is a well-detailed and comprehensive note on how to make fresh fruit salad:

Ingredients:

- Assorted fresh fruits (such as strawberries, blueberries, raspberries, kiwi, pineapple, mango, and grapes)

- Fresh mint leaves

- Lemon juice

Instructions:

1. Wash and prepare the fruits: Rinse the fruits under cold water, pat them dry with a paper towel, and cut them into bite-sized pieces. Remove any stems, seeds, or skins as needed.

2. Combine the fruits: In a large mixing bowl, combine the fruits and gently toss them together.

3. Add fresh mint leaves: Add a handful of fresh mint leaves to the fruit mixture and gently stir to combine.

4. Squeeze lemon juice: Squeeze a fresh lemon over the fruit salad and toss to coat. The

lemon juice will add a zesty, tangy flavor and prevent the fruits from browning.

5. Chill and serve: Cover the bowl with plastic wrap and refrigerate for at least 30 minutes or until ready to serve. Garnish with additional fresh mint leaves before serving.

Serving Suggestions:

- Serve fresh fruit salad as a healthy snack or dessert.

- Top with a dollop of whipped cream or Greek yogurt for added creaminess.

- Drizzle with honey or maple syrup for a touch of sweetness.

- Sprinkle with chopped nuts or granola for added crunch.

Fresh fruit salad is a versatile and delicious dish that can be enjoyed year-round. It's a great way to get your daily dose of vitamins and minerals while satisfying your sweet tooth.

Berry Crisp

Berry Crisp is a delicious and healthy dessert that is perfect for breast cancer patients. It is rich in antioxidants and nutrients, and is made with whole grains, nuts, and fresh berries.

Ingredients:

- 4 cups mixed fresh berries (such as strawberries, blueberries, raspberries, and blackberries)

- 1/4 cup all-purpose flour

- 1/4 cup brown sugar

- 1/2 cup rolled oats

- 1/2 cup chopped pecans or walnuts

- 1/4 cup whole wheat flour

- 1/4 cup butter or coconut oil, softened

- 1 tsp cinnamon

- 1/4 tsp salt

Instructions:

1. Preheat the oven to 375°F.

2. Wash and chop the fresh berries and place them in an 8x8 inch baking dish.

3. In a separate bowl, mix together the all-purpose flour, brown sugar, rolled oats, chopped nuts, whole wheat flour, cinnamon, and salt.

4. Add the softened butter or coconut oil to the mixture and mix well until it forms a crumbly texture.

5. Sprinkle the mixture evenly over the berries.

6. Bake the berry crisp for 30-35 minutes, or until the topping is golden brown and the berries are bubbling.

7. Let the berry crisp cool for a few minutes before serving.

Serving suggestion:

Serve the berry crisp warm with a dollop of Greek yogurt or a scoop of vanilla ice cream. It can be enjoyed as a dessert or a healthy breakfast option. It can also be stored in an airtight container in the refrigerator for up to 3 days.

Oatmeal Raisin Cookies

Oatmeal raisin cookies are a delicious and nutritious snack that can be enjoyed by breast cancer patients. These cookies are high in fiber, which helps to regulate blood sugar levels and improve digestion. They also contain heart-healthy oats and antioxidant-rich raisins, making them a great choice for a healthy dessert.

Ingredients:

- 1 cup all-purpose flour
- 1 tsp baking powder
- 1 tsp ground cinnamon
- 1/2 tsp salt

- 1/2 cup unsalted butter, softened
- 1/2 cup granulated sugar
- 1/2 cup light brown sugar, packed
- 2 large eggs
- 1 tsp vanilla extract
- 1 1/2 cups old-fashioned oats
- 1 cup raisins

Instructions:

1. Preheat the oven to 350°F (175°C) and line a baking sheet with parchment paper.

2. In a medium bowl, whisk together the flour, baking powder, cinnamon, and salt.

3. In a large bowl, cream together the butter, granulated sugar, and brown sugar until light and fluffy, about 2-3 minutes.

4. Beat in the eggs, one at a time, and then the vanilla extract.

5. Gradually stir in the flour mixture, followed by the oats and raisins, until well combined.

6. Drop spoonfuls of dough onto the prepared baking sheet, spacing them about 2 inches apart.

7. Bake for 12-15 minutes, or until the cookies are golden brown.

8. Remove from the oven and let cool on the baking sheet for 5 minutes before transferring to a wire rack to cool completely.

Serving: This recipe makes about 2 dozen cookies. Serve them warm or at room temperature as a healthy and delicious snack or dessert. They can be stored in an airtight container at room temperature for up to 5 days.

Chapter 15

Bonus Resources

• Guide to Breast Cancer Nutrition

Breast cancer is a complex disease, and there are many factors that can impact its development, progression, and treatment.

One area that has received increasing attention in recent years is the role of nutrition in breast cancer management.

Proper nutrition is critical for supporting the immune system, managing side effects of treatment, and potentially even reducing the risk of recurrence.

Here are some key elements of breast cancer nutrition to keep in mind:

1. *A Balanced Diet*: Eating a balanced diet that includes a variety of fruits, vegetables, whole grains, lean proteins, and healthy fats is important for overall health and well-being. A balanced diet can also help to maintain a healthy weight, which is important because obesity has been linked to an increased risk of breast cancer.

2. *Antioxidants:* Antioxidants are substances that help to protect cells from damage caused by free radicals, which can contribute to cancer development. Foods that are rich in antioxidants include berries, dark leafy greens, nuts, and seeds.

3. *Omega-3 Fatty Acids:* Omega-3 fatty acids are a type of healthy fat that has been shown to have anti-inflammatory properties, which may help to reduce the risk of breast cancer. Foods that are high in omega-3s include fatty fish (like salmon), flaxseeds, and chia seeds.

4. *Phytochemicals:*
Phytochemicals are naturally occurring compounds found in plants that have been shown to have cancer-fighting properties. Examples include resveratrol (found in grapes and red wine) and curcumin (found in turmeric).

5. *Limit Processed Foods and Sugar:* Processed foods and foods high in sugar have been linked to an increased risk of cancer and other health problems. Limiting these foods can help to promote overall health and well-being.

6. *Hydration:* Drinking plenty of water is important for overall health and well-being, but it is particularly important for breast cancer patients who may experience side effects from treatment that impact hydration.

It is important to work with a registered dietitian or nutritionist who can help to create an individualized nutrition plan that meets your specific needs and goals.

They can help to ensure that you are getting the nutrients that you need to support your health and well-being, while also managing any side effects of treatment.

Pantry Essentials Checklist

When going through breast cancer treatment, it's important to stock your pantry with healthy and nutritious foods to support your body's healing process. Here's a checklist of pantry essentials for breast cancer patients:

1. *Whole grains*: Brown rice, quinoa, whole wheat pasta, and oats are great sources of fiber and complex carbohydrates.

2. *Legumes:* Lentils, chickpeas, and beans are high in protein, fiber, and other nutrients.

3. *Nuts and seeds:* Almonds, walnuts, chia seeds, and flaxseeds are great sources of healthy fats and protein.

4. *Canned fish:* Canned salmon and tuna are great sources of protein and omega-3 fatty acids.

5. *Vegetables*: Stock up on canned or frozen vegetables like green beans, spinach, broccoli, and carrots for easy meal prep.

6. *Fruits:* Canned or dried fruits like peaches, pears, and apricots are great for snacking or adding to oatmeal and yogurt.

7. *Low-sugar snacks:* Keep some low-sugar snacks on hand like whole grain crackers, rice cakes, or popcorn.

8. Cooking oils: Opt for healthy oils like olive oil, coconut oil, or avocado oil for cooking and baking.

9. Spices and seasonings: Keep a variety of spices and seasonings on hand to add flavor to meals without relying on salt.

By stocking up on these pantry essentials, you'll have the foundation for creating healthy and nourishing meals and snacks throughout your breast cancer journey.

• Meal Planning Tips and Tricks

Meal planning is a crucial aspect of maintaining a healthy diet, especially for breast cancer patients. Here are some tips and tricks for meal planning for breast cancer patients:

1. Plan ahead: Spend some time each week planning your meals and snacks. This will help you make healthier choices and avoid the temptation to grab unhealthy options.

2. Choose nutrient-dense foods: Opt for foods that are high in nutrients and low in calories. These include fruits, vegetables,

whole grains, lean proteins, and healthy fats.

3. Incorporate a variety of colors: Eating a colorful variety of fruits and vegetables ensures that you are getting a wide range of nutrients.

4. Balance your meals: Aim to have a balance of protein, carbohydrates, and healthy fats at each meal.

5. Cook at home: Cooking at home allows you to control the ingredients and avoid added sugars, salt, and unhealthy fats.

6. Use healthy cooking methods: Choose healthy cooking methods like grilling, baking, or steaming instead of frying.

7. Include healthy snacks: Keep healthy snacks like fruits, vegetables, and nuts on hand to help you avoid reaching for unhealthy options.

8. Stay hydrated: Drink plenty of water throughout the day to stay hydrated and help your body function properly.

By following these tips and tricks, you can create a meal plan that supports your health and well-being during and after breast cancer treatment.

• Kitchen Equipment Recommendations

Breast cancer patients may find it helpful to have certain kitchen equipment to aid in meal preparation and cooking. Here are some recommendations:

1. Blender or food processor: A blender or food processor can be used to make smoothies, soups, and sauces that are easy to digest and can help meet nutritional needs.

2. Slow cooker: A slow cooker is a great option for preparing stews, soups, and chili. It allows for easy meal preparation and can be set to cook all day, providing a warm, comforting meal at the end of the day.

3. Steamer basket: A steamer basket can be used to cook vegetables without losing their

nutrients. It is also a healthier cooking option, as it does not require added oils or fats.

4. Non-stick cookware: Non-stick cookware is easier to clean and requires less oil or butter for cooking. This can be especially helpful for those experiencing digestive issues.

5. Sharp knives: Sharp knives can make meal preparation easier and safer. They also require less effort to cut through fruits, vegetables, and meat.

6. Measuring cups and spoons: Measuring cups and spoons are essential for following recipes and ensuring accurate portion sizes.

7. Food storage containers: Having food storage containers on hand can make meal prep and storage easier. Glass or BPA-free plastic containers are recommended.

By having these kitchen equipment on hand, breast cancer patients can make meal preparation and cooking easier and more enjoyable.